ALTERNATIVE MEDICINE WORKS!

Your Primer on Natural Medicine

AJAY GOEL, PH.D., AGAF
AND TERRY LEMEROND

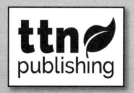

Published by:
Terry Talks Nutrition Publishing
GREEN BAY, WI

Library of Congress Cataloging-in-Publication Data is on file with the Library of Congress.

ISBN: 978-1-952507-60-1

Editor: Kathleen Barnes
Design: Gary A. Rosenberg • www.thebookcouple.com

Printed in the United States of America

10   9   8   7   6   5   4   3   2   1

Contents

SECTION 1

Introduction

From Dr. Ajay Goel and Terry Lemerond

The purpose of this book is not only to educate you but to help educate your doctor.

If you've picked up this book, you've undoubtedly added one or more alternative therapies to your life. Have you ever taken a nutritional supplement? Had a massage? Seen a chiropractor? Meditated? Taken a yoga class?

Congratulations! You're already a part of the alternative medicine world.

Call it alternative medicine, holistic, natural, complementary or something else, this book is designed to help provide answers to chronic health challenges and give you a roadmap along the path to a healthier life.

By way of introductions:

Dr. Goel

Dynamic and passionate—with a formidable record of patented innovations in cancer care—Ajay Goel, Ph.D., AGAF, is committed to developing better methods for the early detection and precision treatment of cancer. He joined City of Hope in June 2019 as the founding chair of the new Department of Molecular Diagnostics and Experimental Therapeutics and founding director of Biotech Innovations at Beckman Research Institute.

A noted expert in gastrointestinal and other cancers, Dr. Goel is currently developing early-detection blood tests for colon, pancreatic and ovarian cancers and a test for pancreatic cancer that can detect the disease seven years earlier than is now possible. Within the next few years, these tests are expected to become a simple and affordable part of everyone's annual health physical, just like tests for diabetes or cholesterol.

He is also working with genomic-based precision oncology to provide answers to the question: Why do therapies work with some good candidates and not with others?

Dr. Goel was born in India. He received his Ph.D. in biophysics from Punjab University, completed his postgraduate work at the University of California, San Diego, and went on to a noteworthy 16-year career at Baylor Scott & White Research Institute in Texas. He has authored more than 425 articles in peer-reviewed international journals and holds more than 60 advanced genomic and transcriptomic international patents.

Dr. Goel is a member of the American Association for Cancer Research and the American Gastroenterology Association and is on the international editorial boards of more than 75 international journals, including *Gastroenterology, Clinical Cancer Research, Molecular Therapy Oncolytics, Digestive Diseases and Sciences, Carcinogenesis,* and *Alternative Therapies in Health and Medicine.* He also performs peer-reviewing activities for almost 125 scientific journals, as well as serves on various grant-funding committees of the National Institutes of Health, the Department of Defense, and more than 50 national and international research foundations.

Terry Lemerond

Terry Lemerond is a natural health expert with over 55 years of experience. He has owned health food stores, founded dietary supplement companies, and formulated over 500 products to help people live healthier lives. A much sought-after speaker and accomplished author, Terry shares his wealth of experience and knowledge in health and nutrition through social media, newsletters, podcasts, webinars, and personal speaking engagements. His books include *Seven Keys to Vibrant Health, Seven Keys to Unlimited Personal Achievement, 50+ Natural Health Secrets Proven to Change Your Life*, and his newest publication, *Discovering Your Best Health – How to Improve Your Health at Any Age.* Terry's weekly radio program, *Terry Talks Nutrition*, airs locally in Green Bay, Wisconsin Saturday and Sunday mornings at 8:00 a.m. CST, and is available online through his educational website at TerryTalksNutrition.com. His continual dedication, energy, and zeal are part of his ongoing mission—to improve the health of America.

Their combined decades of research and experience make Ajay and Terry your best possible guides in the field of alternative medicine.

Welcome to your journey to natural health!

CHAPTER 1

What Is
Alternative Medicine?

Arose by any other name: There are countless variations on the theme of alternatives to conventional medicine.

Let's start with a fundamental definition: We're enthusiastic proponents of natural medicine. That's admittedly an inclusive term. If that sounds vague, read on. In the coming chapters, you'll get a broader view of the various types of natural medicine and concrete examples of how they differ from or are complementary to treatments offered by conventional medicine.

In this book, you'll also learn how modern science is now validating, sometimes enthusiastically, natural treatments for countless illnesses, diseases and maladies that traditional medicine has known and practiced for millennia.

What do we mean by conventional medicine?

It's the type of treatment you would typically receive at your local pharmacy, doctor's office, urgent care or in your local hospital. Sometimes it's called "orthodox" medicine instead of "unorthodox" alternatives.

Let's look at one example: If you seek treatment for the flu, your doctor will likely prescribe Tamiflu, an antiviral medication that, in rare cases, can cause a life-threatening reaction called Stevens-Johnson syndrome.

Treating the flu is a complicated decision for all healthcare practitioners, but getting over the flu fast may not be the wisest choice for you.

For example, the doctor needs to consider your overall general health. An excellent challenge to your immune system might make you stronger. A few days of rest and extra fluids may be enough. Or not.

Perhaps a botanical like melatonin, olive leaf extract, elderberry or even vitamin C would make you feel better without any severe side effects.

We're not here to bash conventional medicine, but we can say that conventionally trained doctors often fail to look at natural remedies that cause few side effects and can improve your overall health.

So, what *is* alternative medicine?

That's a big question! There are as many differing opinions of what the term means as the day is long, so let us offer our opinion as a starting point:

Alternative medicine is a natural medicine that places emphasis on treating the entire human being, body, mind and spirit, not just a disease. Alternative medicine may include a wide range of natural treatment modalities, including dietary solutions, acupuncture, energy medicine, meditation, botanical medicines and much more.

Contrary to some definitions you might find in a Google search, alternative medicine doesn't reject conventional medicine. Conventional medicine has its place. Dr. Andrew Weil, one of the founders of the alternative health movement in America, has oft been quoted, "If I'm in a car accident with a traumatic brain injury, please don't take me to an herbalist."

Yes, there is no doubt that conventional medicine can save lives, especially in cases of severe injuries.

Have you ever been in a hospital? We probably don't need to tell you about the horrors of hospital food! So, what if you'd been in that hypothetical car accident? Surely a healthy, whole-food organic diet will help your body to heal. Perhaps meditation and yoga might help overcome the trauma and improve body mobility. Certain supplements would address pain, promote healing and minimize or eliminate the need for dangerous prescription meds.

The times they are a changin' as Bob Dylan says. In an article about Dr. Andrew Weil way back in 1997, the *New York Times* wrote that we have an "...especially valuable little window of opportunity to convince doctors that alternative medicine really works and to convince the rest of us it isn't kooky. Already yoga seems as normal as aerobics. So, who knows: It may soon seem the most ordinary thing in the world to, say, have your energy channeled during surgery or to leave your pharmacy carrying a box full of plants."

Today, many conventional medical practitioners embrace alternatives. That's good news. Just as many will probably pooh-pooh suggestions that botanicals have healing power that can complement or even replace pharmaceuticals.

But what's even more important is to prevent the disease altogether. We have the tools to do so. Most came from our ancestors who lived simple active lives based on healthy natural diets rich in locally grown fruits and vegetables, pleasurable exercise, nurturing family relationships and fulfilling work.

Uncle Sam buys into alternative medicine.

The U.S. government even embraced at least some of the concepts of alternative and natural medicine when it created the Office of

Alternative Medicine (OAM) in 1991 "to facilitate study and evaluation of complementary and alternative medical practices and to disseminate the resulting information to the public."

In 1998, OAM morphed into NCCAM, the National Center for Complementary and Alternative Medicine under the National Institutes of Health. As attitudes began to change, the term "alternative" was dropped in 2014 when NCCAM was renamed the National Center for Complementary and Integrative Health (NCCIH). This reflects changing attitudes that alternative therapies can complement conventional medicine and even become integrated into standard medical treatment.

NCCIH has contributed significantly to our knowledge of how all forms of medicine can be combined to promote the healing of the entire body.

Among them:

➢ The creation of *HerbList* in 2018, providing science-based information on herbal healing;

➢ Also in 2018, NCCIH awarded six research grants to study behavioral interventions for primary or secondary prevention of opioid use disorder or as complements to medication-assisted treatment;

➢ In 2019, announced a $20 million research program for the first projects of the Sound Health Initiative to research the potential of music for treating various conditions resulting from neurological and other disorders;

➢ In 2020, announced a broad initiative to study alternative treatments for chronic pain and opioid abuse.

➢ And much more.

This is just a long way of saying that alternative, complementary, integrative medicine—whatever you choose to call it—has lost its "kooky" vibe and become an accepted and even respected means of healing.

We dare say that we are on the verge of arriving at a meeting of minds (and bodies) marrying ancient remedies with modern medicine. The result will be healthier, happier and longer lives for all of us.

CHAPTER 2

Botanicals

Plants are at the heart of modern civilization. Thousands of years ago, primitive people keenly observed the natural world and learned about their surroundings. They derived food, clothing, shelter and every type of medicine from plants. Our ancestors quite literally would not have survived without their alliance with the plant world. It's not a stretch to say that life in today's world evolved from plants.

The earliest forms of medicine known to mankind were, without exception, derived from plants. That fundamental truth continues to this day, even though modern medicine attempts to isolate plant parts to create pharmaceutical drugs that can create more problems than they solve. We'll look more deeply at this modern misconception in Chapter 3.

Ancient medicine women and men revered their herbal allies. They knew that the right plant in the correct dosages could halt an asthma attack, support a failing heart, stop bleeding, prevent infections, help heal broken bones and so much more. They also knew that plant medicine could prevent a host of health challenges, so plants were simply a part of their people's daily lives.

Plants were harvested, dug, consumed fresh, dried, extracted, distilled, tinctured and preserved in a broad range of natural ways to access their healing properties whenever needed, regardless of the season.

Botanical or herb?

Botanical or herb? We say po-tay-to, you say po-tah-to. Technically, a botanical is a blanket term for anything made from plant material. This includes plants, as we generally define them, fungi (mushrooms), rhizomes (roots), algae, bark, twigs, berries and other plant parts. Botanicals are available as teas, infusions, creams, essential oils and supplements in capsule, tablet or powder form.

An herb is defined as leaves stems, flowers or other aboveground plant parts that can be used for healing or nutritional purposes.

We can add spices to this botanical mix as well. Spices are used for flavoring foods, perfume and cosmetics, whether or not they have any specific medicinal value.

Here's a great example: Dr. Goel has extensively researched curcumin, especially its preventive and curative effects against

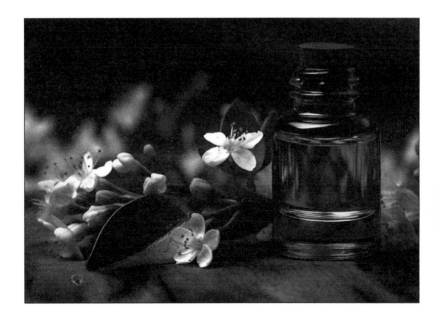

various types of cancer. Curcumin and turmeric are derivatives of the same *Curcuma longa* plant, but "turmeric is the spice (that gives Indian curries their typical yellow color and flavor), and curcumin is the medicine."

We don't have to split hairs here. Can we agree that botanicals are healing plants?

Botanicals used today can be as simple as wild-crafted rose hips that nearly anyone can gather for teas rich in natural vitamin C to enormously complex medicine compounded from multiple plant sources that may require elaborate steam and alcohol distillation to extract the medicinal compounds.

Healthcare professionals who know about botanicals

Naturopathic doctors undergo training similar to conventional medical doctors: at least four years of training at an accredited naturopathic medical school and passing two licensing exams. A licensed naturopathic doctor, also referred to as naturopathic physician, will carry the initials "ND." Be mindful that there are practitioners who may refer to themselves as "naturopaths," but if they are not licensed NDs, their educational training does not result in a doctorate-level degree.

Not all states recognize naturopathic medicine. Many naturopaths are also trained and, where appropriate, licensed in Traditional Chinese Medicine or Ayurvedic Medicine as well.

Herbalists can be trained in a variety of ways, and most states do not require licensure, but many are highly aware of the positive effects of botanicals.

All of this adds up to the fact that highly trained healthcare professionals understand the value of botanicals and know how to tap plants' healing potential and disease prevention in ways of which most conventional doctors (MDs) are unaware.

Be aware

Be aware that botanicals rarely have an instant effect. There are some exceptions, but most botanicals are slow acting and gentle.

If you have struggled in the past with harsh side effects from using over-the-counter or prescription drugs, a botanical medicine may be a better choice for you.

If you are taking a botanical, please give it at least a month and preferably two months for it to build in your system and take effect.

What's on today's market

Luckily, you don't have to roam the woods to wildcraft ginseng, become a scuba diver to harvest seaweed, or travel to India to reap the best curcumin. Virtually every botanical medicine is freely available on the market today. You can get anything you need at your local health food store, including expert advice.

However, it's essential to research any botanical supplements, even teas, that you are considering as the regulations regarding the sale of natural herbs and botanicals are different from the rules for prescription and over-the-counter medications. As a consumer, you may have to put in a little more detective work to identify reputable products.

How to choose the best botanical product

Caveat emptor (buyer beware):

➢ Most botanicals are extracted from the plant material using water, steam, or alcohol as solvents. However, some botanicals are extracted with toxic and cancer-causing chemicals like benzene, carbon tetrachloride and trichloroethylene that can leave harmful residues. Note: Labels won't reflect the use of these types of chemicals. Choose a brand name that you can trust. Read on for ways to determine who is reputable.

➤ Cheapest is usually not the best. Frequently cheaper products have useless fillers and very little, if any, of the advertised plant material. Some even contain illicit pharmaceuticals, animal waste, hair, fungi and unhealthy bacteria. I can remember several years ago, a so-called herbal product being touted for erectile dysfunction actually contained no saw palmetto. This botanical can be helpful and instead contained Viagra, a pharmaceutical that can have fatal side effects for some men.

Take a close look at the label to determine if you can trust a product you are considering:

➤ The botanical name of the ingredients should be included, i.e., Curcumin (*Curcuma longa*);

➤ A list of all active ingredients;

➤ The part of the plant used in the product;

➤ The concentration of the active ingredient(s) in the product;

➤ Recommended serving size;

➤ A detailed description of "other ingredients," including binders, fillers, flavorings, and preservatives. (These aren't necessarily bad, but you need to know, especially if you have severe allergies);

➤ For the same reason as the last point, look for a notification whether the product contains wheat, corn, soy, artificial preservatives or coloring;

➤ The manufacturer's contact information so you can ask questions, if necessary;

➤ Notification of recognized good manufacturing practices, i.e., "manufactured by a cGMP compliant facility;".

➤ An expiration date;

➤ A lot number so the product can be tracked in the case of a recall.

Summing it up...

Plant medicine is the most widely used form of alternative medicine. It brings ancient wisdom to today's medical treatment. In data collected as part of the National Health and Nutrition Examination Survey (pre-COVID), 58.5% of Americans and more than one-third of American children take some form of supplements, many of them derived from plants. It's probably reasonable to project that supplement use increased during the COVID emergency as people sought ways to stay healthy and to address long-COVID.

Botanicals have been the healing choice of people worldwide since time immemorial. Today, plants remain our most valuable healing tools as they have ever been, perhaps even more so now that science has validated their safety and effectiveness.

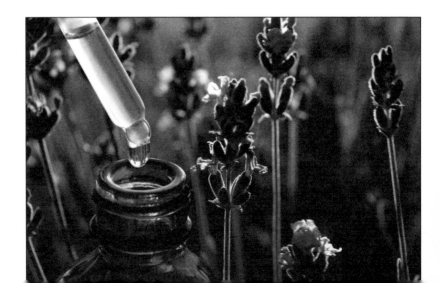

CHAPTER 3

How Pharmaceuticals Are Developed (And Why They Have So Many Negative Side Effects)

Plants are incredibly complex combinations of elements. Modern science has barely begun to investigate the variety of molecules in each seemingly simple plant, much less to understand how each component interacts with the others or affects a broad range of body functions.

In fact, plant components create synergy, meaning that all of those individual parts add up to a health bang for your buck greater than the effects of each individual molecule.

All plants are made up of hundreds of molecules that work on multiple pathways in the body, all simultaneously.

For reasons we cannot understand, drug companies typically create a new drug by isolating one or two tiny elements of a whole plant that might contain thousands of components. Then they present it as a way of addressing complicated medical conditions like cancer or diabetes or heart disease. It simply doesn't work, or if it does work temporarily, it almost inevitably causes terrible side effects.

That, in a nutshell (pun intended), is what is wrong with how pharmaceutical drugs are formulated today.

We're sure most of you have seen television ads for pharmaceutical drugs that tout how wonderful they are to treat cancer, diabetes, depression, psoriasis, or whatever until they get to the legal disclaimer. They always end with a rapidly talking announcer detailing the dire side effects - that may even include death.

Really? Do you want to take that?

What are pathways?

Let's pause a moment here to take a quick look at pathways as explained by the National Institutes of Health:

From both inside and outside the body, cells are constantly receiving chemical cues prompted by such things as injury, infection, stress or even the presence or lack of food. To react and adjust to these cues, cells send and receive signals through biological pathways. The molecules that make up biological pathways interact with signals, as well as with each other, to carry out their designated tasks.

Biological pathways can act over short or long distances. For example, some cells send signals to nearby cells to repair localized damage, such as a scratch on a knee. Other cells produce substances, such as hormones, that travel through the blood to distant target cells.

These biological pathways control a person's response to the world. For example, some pathways subtly affect how the body processes drugs, while others play a major role in how a fertilized egg develops into a baby. Other pathways maintain balance while a person is walking, control how and when the pupil in the eye opens or closes in response to light and affect the skin's reaction to changing temperature.

Now let's take this explanation of these pathways to the plant world.

Why single-pathway drugs don't work

We mentioned a few pages back that whole plants are made of incredibly complex numbers of substances that communicate with several different types of pathways in the human body and send healing in several directions all at once. That's why botanicals work, and pharmaceuticals frequently don't work.

Dr. Goel offers this example from his cancer research: Pharmaceuticals, especially those that target cancer in various ways, are limited in what they can accomplish since they are composed of one molecule targeting one pathway in the body, thereby throwing many other pathways out of balance.

"Our 2018 work, published in *Scientific Reports*, confirmed the effectiveness of a combination of French grape seed extract and curcumin, particularly its excellent ability to stop tumor formation.

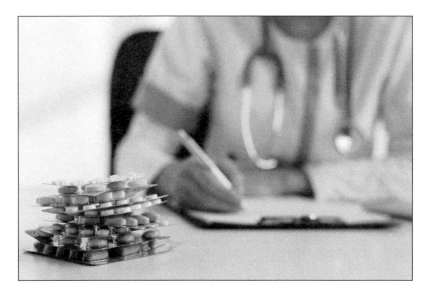

"No pharmaceuticals have these properties, mainly because conventional anti-cancer drugs throw genetic pathways out of balance. They further disrupt homeostasis (balance) and require other drugs to try to bring the body back into balance, creating a vicious circle and a downward spiral that nearly all oncologists acknowledge is part of the progression of cancer.

"We do have such a substance: Our research proves that French grape seed extract and its super medicinal oligomeric proanthocyanins cut off those blood vessels while multi-tasking several other anti-cancer activities.

"In my experience, these natural ingredients can have impressive long-term benefits. They are free from the side effects and complications caused by pharmaceuticals. More and more physicians are beginning to see that the side effects of pharmaceutical drugs often outweigh their benefits."

We think botanicals are like having a pharmacy in a bottle without fearing side effects.

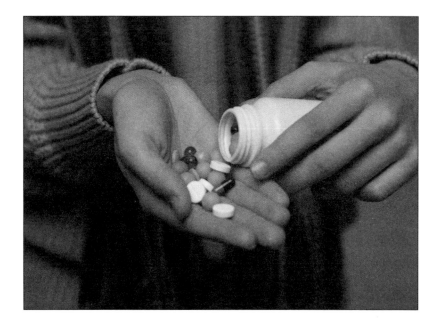

Cost of pharmaceuticals

Yes, of course, there are extremely valuable prescription drugs that have changed the course of human history. The important discoveries of antibiotics, insulin, and vaccines against a host of terrible diseases come immediately to mind as prime examples of Big Pharma wearing a white hat.

But we all know that Big Pharma is highly motivated by profits. That greed, especially in the past couple of decades, has resulted in the opioid pandemic that has cost hundreds of thousands of lives, the skyrocketing costs of insulin and other essential drugs, and hugely expensive cancer drugs that are only marginally effective.

Big Pharma says that the high cost of prescription drugs in the United States is because of the high cost of developing new drugs. The new drug price tag is exponentially exaggerated, according to the international medical crisis non-profit Medicins Sans Frontieres (Doctors Without Borders), which estimates the average cost of developing a new drug is $100-$200 million, less than 10% of the $2-$3 billion cost claimed by Big Pharma.

In conclusion

Now that you have the tools to understand how pharmaceutical drugs are developed and why, we think the answer is clear: botanicals can be a wiser, safer, and more effective ways of treating and preventing health challenges.

CHAPTER 4

How Conventional Medicine Views Alternative Medicine (and Vice Versa)

There are simple and complex answers to this question. Let's start with the simple one:

Here's a simple example:

You've got a cold. It's your fourth this year. Initially, your doctor recommends increased fluids and rest or maybe even a prescription anti-viral drug. . . You don't get better. In a couple of weeks, your doc says you have bronchitis, a bacterial infection, and recommends antibiotics. You get better for a while, and then a couple of months later, another cold hits you, and this time you end up with what your doctor calls "walking pneumonia," also a bacterial infection. You get another round of more potent antibiotics, but your poor body is exhausted and you can't regain your normal vigor.

Conventional medicine treats illnesses and symptoms.
Alternative medicine looks at causes of illness,
prevention of illness and healing for illness in view
of the whole human body, mind and spirit.

What's happened?

Your problem started with a cold, which is a viral infection. It deteriorated into two serious bacterial infections.

Your conventional (or allopathic) doc treated the symptoms with prescription drugs.

On the first visit, with the complaint of your fourth cold this year, an alternative practitioner might have asked if you are under great stress. Do you have extra challenges at work? With your kids or your partner? Financial concerns?

Your "alt doc" is looking at the effects of stress on your entire body and mind. They are working on the fact that unrelieved stress compromises the immune system. A weakened immune system makes you extra vulnerable to viral and bacterial infections.

"Alt doc's" prescription?

➢ Meditation for 10 minutes daily

➢ A 15-minute daily walk to help relieve stress and strengthen your entire organism.

➢ A daily smoothie with lots of nutrient-rich greens and berries.

➢ Immune system strengthening supplements like andrographis, elderberry, curcumin, garlic, and melatonin.

We bet you will never deteriorate to bacterial bronchitis or pneumonia if you treat the underlying causes of your weakened immune system. That's because you've re-set your chronic stress response, strengthened your immune system, and beat the bugs.

If that isn't enough, you may eventually need antibiotics, but they should be the last resort, not the first. We are extremely overexposed to antibiotics in our food and medicines to the point where, for many people, they are ineffective when you need life-saving drugs.

Alternative practitioners

There are several types of alternative medicine practitioners, including:

Osteopathic Doctors (DO)

A DO is the direct holistic counterpart to an allopathic doctor or MD. Both types of doctors must attend an accredited medical school for four years and pass licensing exams. Both can write prescriptions and are licensed to practice in all 50 states. The major difference is the osteopath's focus on prevention and whole-body treatment. Beyond the typical medical curriculum, DOs must complete 200 hours of osteopathic manipulative treatment (OMT) training, learning the science of physically manipulating body tissue to treat patients.

Chiropractic Doctors (DC)

Chiropractic generally employs spinal manipulations to stimulate the body's ability to heal musculoskeletal misalignments and disorders. Chiropractic doctors undergo at least four years of postgraduate training at an accredited college or university and pass state and federal licensing exams. All states license chiropractors, but licensing requirements vary.

Naturopathic Physicians (ND)

Educated and trained in accredited four-year naturopathic medical colleges with similar curriculae to conventional medical schools, naturopathic physicians focus on removing obstacles to the body's innate healing abilities, prevention and holistic treatment of acute and chronic illnesses. An ND's primary healing modalities will be botanicals, including herbs and supplements, but they often use acupuncture, homeopathy, and nutrition for healing. Some states license naturopathic physicians, and some do not. In some states, they can write prescriptions; in others, they cannot.

Herbalists

Herbalists are plant medicine specialists but do not have medical degrees. Most herbalists have certifications in herbal medicine, including a 12-month training course or an associate's degree. Registered herbalists must have 400 hours of clinical experience and 800 hours of classroom experience. However, there are no states that license herbalists. In addition to botanicals, herbalists may also use fungal and bee products, minerals, shells, and sometimes certain animal parts.

Traditional Chinese Medicine (TCM) Doctors (DCM) and Acupuncturists

Doctors of Chinese Medicine undergo specialized training that typically takes five years to complete. The curriculum deeply explores areas of Traditional Chinese Medicine such as psychology, oncology, gerontology, acupuncture, and the classic texts that first recorded the principles of this powerful and ancient system of medicine. While virtually all DCMs have studied and can practice acupuncture, the science of balancing energy meridians often with the use of thin needles, an acupuncturist needs training in other elements of TCM. Most acupuncturists hold at least a master's degree. Some states license both TCMs and acupuncturists, but many do not.

Ayurvedic Doctors and Practitioners

Widely practiced in India, the ancient Ayurvedic tradition promotes balance of body, mind, and spirit. Botanicals play an important role in the prevention-based healing system. There are no specific state licensures in Ayurvedic medicine, so it falls into a gray area of little oversight and ancient wisdom.

Homeopathic Practitioners

The underlying premise of homeopathy is quite similar to the way some vaccines work by giving a tiny dose of the disease-causing substance to a healthy individual to stimulate an immune response. Botanicals are the most common forms of homeopathic remedies concentrated in molecular form. Homeopathic practitioners generally complete a four-year diploma program that includes two years of clinical practice. Only three states offer homeopathic medical licenses.

The good, the bad, and the ugly

The good

Many conventional doctors today endorse, practice, and even personally employ various alternative modalities. While allopathic medicine is focused on treating disease, increasingly, MDs accept certain tenets of holistic medicine and recommend them to their patients.

The bad

We hate to put it this way, but most allopathic doctors need to be made aware of alternative, complementary and integrative medicine and how much they can help prevent illnesses and help their patients heal. For more specifics, see Chapters 5–9.

The ugly

Even more sadly, some MDs, unaware of their own ignorance, hurt their patients by denouncing alternative modalities. Some call them "dangerous" and "quackery." Virtually all of these alternative forms of medicine have been practiced through the centuries, extensively researched in modern times and validated and proven to be effective on their own and in concert with allopathic medicine.

In conclusion, we know from history and science that alternative medicine works. The proof we'll give you in the coming chapters may provide the evidence you'll need if you ever need to convince your conventional doctor to give alternative modalities a chance. They may actually save your life.

SECTION 2

Alternative Specialties

We've already touched on the concepts of alternative medicine, and now it's time to break it down into some subspecialties that have evolved over the years.

Fifty years ago, it was considered "weird" to take supplements. Even if grandma doled out elderberry tincture when you had a cold, it was still "weird."

Yoga was especially weird, even though virtually every YMCA and community center offers yoga classes today.

Acupuncture? Really? Sticking needles under your skin to heal ailments? Yes, really, says the science that originated in China centuries ago, where it is commonly used as an anesthetic and to treat a broad range of illnesses.

Over the years, we've had a national shift in attitudes.

Today, nearly 60% of American adults take at least one supplement and over one-third of children are given supplements.

Meditation, a staple of the comparatively physically and mentally healthy Indian culture, has steadily gained practitioners, with the numbers tripling between 2012 and 2017 to about 15% of the adult population, according to the National Center for

Complementary and Integrative Health. Now meditation is universally recognized for its contribution to stress relief and as a validated way to address heart disease, high blood pressure, anxiety, chronic pain, and depression.

Changing attitudes toward meditation and using botanicals are signs that conventional doctors are gradually integrating alternative thought into their practices. A 2022 review of conventional medical specialists who accepted at least some tenets of complementary and alternative medicine (CAM) rose to 52%, with 45% of specialists adopting at least some CAM strategies in their practices.

In this section, we'll take a little bit deeper dive into the sub-categories of unconventional medicine.

CHAPTER 5

Integrative/ Complementary Medicine

ntegrative and complementary medicine have evolved dramatically over the past couple of decades.

While terminologies vary, some people say that alternative medicine is used *instead* of mainstream medicine, while integrative and complementary medicine are terms that combine and even integrate alternative medicine with conventional medical treatments.

According to the National Institutes of Health's National Center for Complementary and Integrative Health (NCCIH), "The terms "complementary," "alternative," and "integrative" are continually evolving." About 30% of American adults use health care approaches "that are not typically part of conventional medical care or that may have origins outside of usual Western practice," noting that most people who use non-conventional forms of medical care also use conventional health care.

The terms "integrative" and "complementary" are interchangeable for the most part when we look at the ways conventional and holistic medical techniques can enhance one another.

In the best of all worlds, the practices of Western medicine that often emphasize pharmaceuticals, surgery and invasive treatments are now frequently combined with complementary or integrative therapies like botanicals, yoga, acupuncture., psychological therapies and more with a focus on treating the whole person rather than just one organ system.

For example, cancer doctors might now quite commonly offer nutritional counseling to their patients and perhaps add supplements known to enhance traditional treatment like chemotherapy, with acupuncture for pain management and perhaps meditation to reduce stress. Conventional cancer care usually includes surgery, chemotherapy and sometimes radiation. All of these have serious and sometimes fatal side effects, so conventional doctors are increasingly open to integrative treatments. Some are even enthusiastic supporters of botanicals that can help improve the effectiveness of chemotherapy while protecting healthy tissues. Some who have taken the time to educate themselves are embracing long-term use of botanicals that prevent cancer from recurring, all without serious side effects. (See more detailed explanation about proven positive effects of botanicals in Chapter 9.)

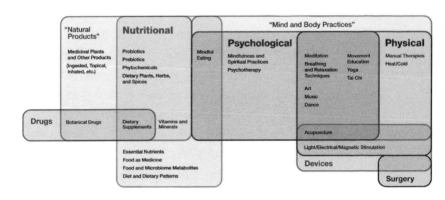

(credit: NCCIH)

Botanicals

Nearly 60% of American adults use supplements, which are by far the most popular complementary health approach.

Since both of us have researched botanicals for five decades, plant medicine is clearly close to my heart. It is such a joy to us that "modern" medicine is finally catching up with the wisdom of our ancestors! We think it's even more gratifying when we hear how patients are enlightening their doctors and persuading them to embrace integrative practices.

We dare say the rise of the Internet has empowered many of us as consumers of medical services to press our doctors to open their minds and look into alternatives to invasive and sometimes toxic approaches.

Plant medicine works. There is ample proof of it in the form of literally millions of studies published in modern peer-reviewed medical journals. The U.S. government and governments around the world have invested in agencies to research and validate or reject a host of complementary and integrative approaches.

Modern day validation of botanical medicine is so important that I'm devoting an entire chapter to it (Chapter 9). Please read on!

Other complementary and integrative approaches

When was the last time your doctor suggested that a safe and effective curcumin supplement might help relieve your joint pain instead of a prescription drug that has serious side effects, including causing heart attacks and strokes? Or has your doctor suggested that aiming for nine servings of fruits and vegetables daily are proven to give you a longer healthier life? Or maybe you've gotten a referral to a massage therapist to help correct your lower back pain? Believe me, it's happening every day! We are all better for it.

Let's take a look at other complementary and integrative therapies and the modern-day view of their effectiveness.

Research findings confirm that psychological and physical approaches, alone or in combination, are helpful for a variety of conditions.

There are probably hundreds of complementary and integrative therapies and their variations. Here's a quick look at just a few of the best-known ones:

Yoga: As we mentioned at the beginning of this chapter, a few decades ago, yoga was considered "weird," but now the ancient Indian practice of conscious movement, breathing exercises and meditation is everywhere for a multitude of good reasons.

More than 7,500 studies confirm that yoga improves general wellness by relieving stress, supporting good health habits, promoting healing sleep, improving mental/emotional health, balance, menopause symptoms, memory and mental clarity. Yoga also eases low-back pain and neck pain, anxiety, depression, quitting smoking and helps improve quality of life for people with chronic diseases.

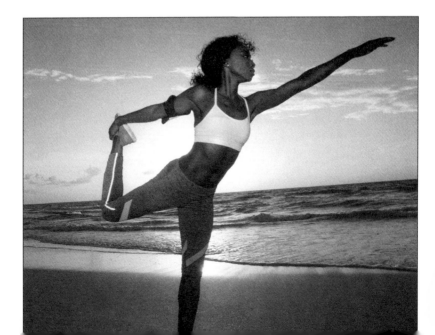

According to the 2017 US National Health Interview Survey conducted by the National Institutes of Health, the popularity of yoga has grown dramatically in recent years, from 9.5 percent of U.S. adults practicing yoga in 2012 to 14.3 percent in 2017. The 2017 NHIS also showed that the use of meditation increased more than threefold from 4.1 percent in 2012 to 14.2 percent in 2017.

Acupuncture: This Chinese treatment that focuses on healing through stimulation of energy meridians in the body, has been used for at least 2,500 years. It's most frequently used to address painful musculoskeletal injuries and chronic pain, including low-back, neck and osteo-arthritis/knee pain. It's also often used to treat a variety of types of headaches, including migraines, menopausal symptoms, nausea, depression and treatment of addiction, including smoking. Acupuncture famously has been used as an anesthetic during abdominal surgeries with no pain to the patient, 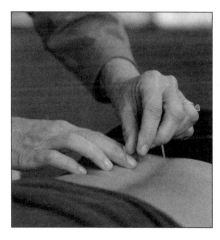 continuing postsurgical pain relief and faster wound healing.

The National Library of Medicine's database has more than 41,000 published studies on acupuncture, 6,550 of them clinical trials on human patients. This again confirms the effectiveness and safety of another ancient form of medicine.

Chiropractic: As mentioned, in the past chapters, chiropractors are licensed medical professionals who undergo training similar to medical doctors with an extra emphasis on correction of musculoskeletal imbalances through manipulation of the spine. Every state in the US licenses chiropractors.

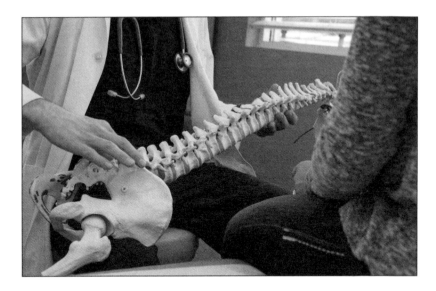

Chiropractic has long been an accepted medical treatment, one of the few complementary and integrative treatments covered by most insurance plans.

The spinal adjustments made by chiropractors increase blood flow and nerve conductivity to the joints to promote healing of injuries as well as correcting spine and joint misalignments.

While some conventional doctors may disagree on the benefits of chiropractic, there is a wealth of evidence that chiropractic adjustments can ease pain, particularly back pain.

Meditation: There are dozens, perhaps hundreds, of forms of meditation ranging from the stereotypical quiet practitioner sitting in the lotus posture to wild ecstatic trance dance and just about everything you can imagine in between.

While meditation is most often practiced to relieve stress, more than 1,300 published studies show it can also relieve anxiety disorder and clinically diagnosed depression, lower blood pressure, improve immune function and balance, reduce symptoms of ADHD, insomnia, gastrointestinal disorders and much more.

In our stressful world, meditation has become a useful life balancing tool for an estimated 275 million practitioners worldwide, about 15% of them in the U.S. It is the most widely used non-supplement form of complementary and alternative medicine.

Mindfulness meditation focuses on awareness of what you're feeling or sensing in the moment without judgment. It usually involves breathing techniques and sometimes guided imagery and progressive relaxation techniques. Meditation apps have become increasingly popular in recent years.

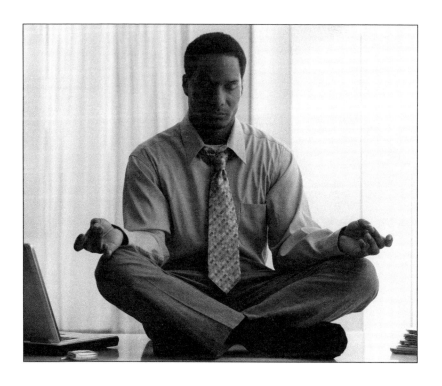

TEN MOST COMMON COMPLEMENTARY HEALTH APPROACHES AMONG ADULTS

Natural Products* 17.7%

Deep Breathing 10.9%

Yoga, Tai Chi, or Qi Gong 10.1%

Chiropractic or Osteopathic Manipulation. 8.4%

Meditation. 6.9%

Special Diets 3.0%

Homeopathy 2.2%

Progressive Relaxation. 2.1%

Guided Imagery 1.7%

*Dietary supplements other than vitamins and minerals.

Source: Clarke TC, Black LI, Stussman BJ, Barnes PM, Nahin RL. Trends in the use of complementary health approaches among adults: United States, 2002–2012. National health statistics reports; no 79. Hyattsville, MD: National Center for Health Statistics. 2015.

CHAPTER 6

Functional Medicine

Functional medicine goes a step farther than integrative and complementary medicine. While functional medicine is often an approach to chronic diseases, anyone can benefit from this approach that we think of as "whole-istic."

Functional medicine is based on dual underlying approaches:

1. The need to identify and address the root cause of disease;

2. The concept that each person and each health challenge is individual and each should be addressed for the unique needs of that individual and that specific disease, a concept called "bio-individuality" rather than conventional medicine's approach to treating symptoms.

Our understanding of the disease process and its causes is evolving as science evolves. This has resulted in dramatic changes to how we and our healthcare professionals view the disease process, in many cases leading to far more successful treatments.

Functional medicine investigates symptoms, not seeking to silence them, but to find and treat the underlying cause.

For example, if you're feeling depressed, there could be a number of underlying causes. You might have a nutritional deficiency or low thyroid function, or you might have pre-diabetes. Instead of simply prescribing an anti-depressant drug as

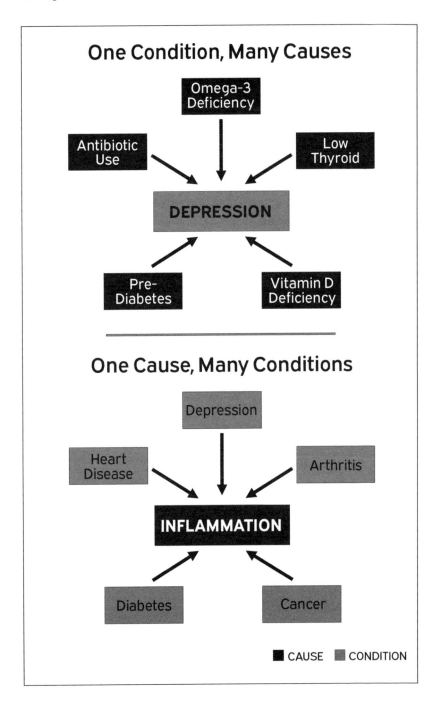

conventional doctors are likely to, a functional medicine doctor will ask you LOTS of questions, do the medical tests necessary to find the cause of your depression, and find the proper treatment for you.

Conversely, we know chronic inflammation is an underlying cause of many diseases. So, if you have heart disease, diabetes, arthritis, or even cancer, your functional medicine clinician will look at the cause of the inflammation. Those causes might include an autoimmune disorder, toxic exposure, obesity or an untreated acute inflammation like you might find with an infection or an injury.

How does your doctor know if you have chronic inflammation? A blood test measures a protein produced by the liver, C-reactive protein (CRP), which rises in response to inflammation. A CRP level between 1 and 3 mg per liter of blood often signals a low, yet chronic, level of inflammation.

Your functional medicine provider is a detective. By taking that deeper dive into your health situation, you have a far better chance of getting the right answers and the treatment that will be the most effective for you.

Timeline

All doctors take a patient's medical history. Of course, a functional medicine practitioner will want to know your medical history. In the case of functional medicine, that medical history will be much more detailed. The Timeline also includes family medical history, personal health and lifestyle history, medical symptoms, diet, exercise patterns, and traumas.

The Institute of Functional Medicine explains:

"What makes the Timeline different than other tools is that it has the effect of giving the patient insight into previous life

events and validates for them that their story has been heard,
both of which help to motivate them to make lifestyle modifica-
tions and engage more fully in the treatment plan. The Timeline
is patient-centered because it places central importance on the
patient's experience, not just the clinician's interpretation of the
patient's symptoms."

In short terms, this means the clinician will spend quite a bit of
time with you (what a welcome element that is!), not only getting
to know about your health issues but getting to know you—that
bio-individual "you" that will help you get a complete diagnosis
based on all of the elements of your life. This is a critical tool in
uncovering the underlying causes of your unique health profile.

Four Pillars of Functional Medicine

1. **Movement:** If you choose a functional medicine practitioner,
   expect to be asked about your exercise program and have your
   muscular strength, endurance, and flexibility tested. They'll
   also want to look at your posture.

2. **Nutrition:** You'll also be asked detailed questions about your
   eating habits, the types of foods you eat, and your caloric intake.
   They'll want to know what supplement you take, and they can
   advise you on supplements, particularly botanicals, that will
   help address your individual health challenges.

3. **Stress Management:** They'll want to know what you do for self-
   care. Meditation? Other stress management techniques. If you
   don't have such tools, your functional medicine provider will
   offer them.

4. **Community:** You'll be asked if you have a close relationship
   with nearby family and friends. How do you connect with yourself? Do you spend time in nature?

The above four points are called the Four Pillars of Functional Medicine. They are key to your partnership with your functional healthcare provider that will help result in a healthier, happier lifestyle and possible reversal of the chronic disease.

Who are functional medicine practitioners?

They are already highly educated healthcare professionals.

In order to have a post-graduate certification in functional medicine, these practitioners must already have at least an undergraduate degree in some area of health care. Many are M.D.s or D.O.s. Chiropractors, naturopathic doctors, pharmacists, mental health professionals, dentists, nurse practitioners, physician assistants, registered nurses, registered dietitians, and occupational and physical therapists can all obtain these additional functional medicine certifications.

Increasing numbers of conventional doctors are feeling frustrated with today's severe limitations on doctor time with patients and increasing emphasis on "the bottom line," profit over true health care. That's why approximately 20% of primary care physicians in the U.S. have received additional training in functional and integrative techniques.

Many functional medical practices will include several types of practitioners to address the "whole you." These may include nutrition counseling, mental health counseling, exercise coaches, massage therapists, and more.

If you've been on a long journey, you're struggling to understand your health issues, a functional medicine health care professional may help you find answers.

CHAPTER 7

Precision Medicine

Precision medicine, sometimes called "personalized" medicine has simple and easily understandable applications as well as incredibly complex ones.

In the simplest terms, precision medicine takes a look at the entire individual in terms of age, gender, lifestyle and genetics when making prevention and treatment decisions.

Rejecting the idea of "one size fits all" medicine isn't new. In fact, Sir William Osler, MD, (1849-1919) one of the founders of Johns Hopkins Hospital, is generally recognized as the founder of the concept: "It is much more important to know what sort of a patient has a disease than what sort of a disease a patient has."

In today's terms, precision medicine is largely reliant on genetic information in ways that were unthinkable a couple of decades ago to create individualized treatment plans to treat and prevent many types of diseases.

The National Cancer Institute applauds the emergence of what is often called "bioindividualized" medicine:

"Historically, doctors have had to make most recommendations about disease prevention and treatment based on the *expected* (emphasis ours) response of an average patient. This one-size-fits-all approach works well for some patients and some conditions, but not so much for others.

"Precision medicine is an innovative approach that takes into account individual differences in patients' genes, environments and lifestyles. Millions of people have already been touched by the area of precision medicine that has grown directly from biomedical research."

In the past (and sometimes still today), doctors would use a shotgun approach to diseases, especially cancer, throwing a battery of harmful drugs at each patient in hopes that something would work. Today we can find solutions with great precision, hence the name "precision" medicine. Interestingly, we can also find out what *doesn't* work and why.

Since about the beginning of the 21st century when we began to decipher DNA, we now have immeasurably deeper insights into genetics. Precision medicine has given us unprecedented opportunities to match the right treatments to the right people based on the genetic makeup of their disease or their risk for disease based on genetic factors

Doctors can now take a sample of a cancerous tumor and by analyzing its genetic makeup, be able to create a treatment plan that will have far greater chances of success based on that individual's unique genetic makeup.

Genetic information can also predict the likelihood of an individual developing breast cancer or Alzheimer's disease or any of a huge range of inherited diseases.

Precision medicine is actually the penultimate description of "holistic" medicine in which the entire organism is taken into consideration when devising treatment and prevention plans.

Precision medicine and cancer

Cancer research, Dr. Goel's specialty, is at the forefront of precision medicine.

From Dr. Goel:

Cancer is a terribly complex disease. The "oldthink" of treating every type of cancer identically with standardized treatments failed because cancer cells are smart. They're so smart that they almost seem to have a brain of their own. As soon as we target cancer cells from one direction, they change direction and become resistant to whatever therapy worked last week or last month.

I have been researching cancer for nearly 30 years. I can say unequivocally that cancer is a different disease in every single case.

I've long advocated deep analysis of individual cancerous tumors. This quantum leap in our ability to analyze each person's tumor on the genetic and molecular levels also allows us to devise very specific custom-tailored, precision medicine plans for each patient.

To successfully treat cancer, we must first understand the individual nature of each person's cancer. Then we must approach that cancer from a wide variety of ways. We need to *see* what will work this week and *anticipate* what will work next week. What will work in the future course of an individual's disease will assuredly be different than what has worked in the past.

Yes, there are commonalities, but cancer evolves through a complex roadmap of genes and pathways that can take on exponential numbers of possibilities. Therefore, we need to approach it knowing that those smart cancer cells can adapt to the ever-evolving disease in each cancer patient with an impressive speed.

Therefore, we must pivot in our thinking and learn lessons from modern science, which tells us that 'targeted' cancer treatments (against a single gene or pathway) that we have been using for the past two decades are only going to help the small group of patients who have early-stage cancers.

For most of our patients, we must use a multipronged approach that is broader and benefits from a 'multi-targeted' plan that can simultaneously target multiple genes and pathways, assure improved quality of life, reduced chances of cancer relapse and prolonged healthy life. This is something modern medicine currently lacks.

In the past 30 years, science has unlocked a vast amount of information that helps us prevent, diagnose and treat cancer and other diseases. Genetic analysis has made it possible for us to analyze the exact cellular components of cancerous cells from each patient and determine, project and confirm what will work for that specific disease.

The Genome Project, a cooperative international scientific exploration, set out to map the entire human DNA sequence in 1990. The results reported in 2003 mapped 90% of the human genome, enormously changing medicine and our understanding of the human body. In the intervening 20 years, this knowledge has continued to evolve at a rapid pace. In 2022, the Telomere to Telomere Consortium announced it had filled in the gaps and successfully mapped 100% of the human genome.

These advances have opened the doors to targeted treatment for a wide variety of diseases and, perhaps more importantly, to identify people with genetic risk factors so preventive measures can be taken before the disease occurs.

When we add exercise, diet, environment and other lifestyle factors, we have a truly impressive arsenal to prevent and fight a wide range of diseases, not just cancer.

CHAPTER 8

Ayurveda and Chinese Medicine

These two ancient and deeply revered medical traditions deserve a deeper exploration here because they are foundational to many of today's alternatives to conventional medicine. They are the world's oldest medical traditions.

They are truly "traditional" medicine since both have been practiced for thousands of years in India and China.

Ayurveda

This 5,000-year-old whole-body tradition is still widely practiced in India. Taken from the Sanskrit words that mean "the science of life," Ayurveda promotes balance of body, mind and spirit and is the premise that underlies Western holistic medicine.

From the Ayurvedic viewpoint, disease comes from imbalances in body, mind and/or spirit.

Promoting the flow of *prana*, the body's natural energy and life force, Ayurvedic practitioners rely on three generalized body types called doshas that govern the way the entire body should be treated. Does that sound like precision medicine? It is an ancient form of medical treatment that is still practiced effectively today.

Three doshas

Ayurveda is based on a complex system of body typing that begins with the five elements of ether, air, fire, water, and earth. The unique combination of all five of these come together to comprise the doshas.

While most of us have one dominant dosha (if you read below, you'll probably identify yourself quite easily), we also have a secondary and the third would be the least prominent. Treatment of illness depends in an individual's dosha and almost invariably includes dietary recommendations, lifestyle changes, natural supplementation often with botanicals, yoga and meditation.

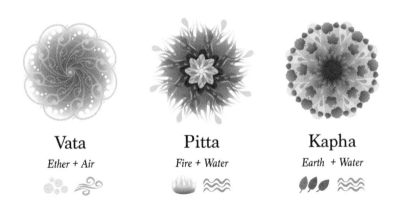

Vata	Pitta	Kapha
Ether + Air	*Fire + Water*	*Earth + Water*

This is a very basic description of the body types that are dominant in each dosha:

Vata, the air dosha: People with dominant vata tend to be thin and energetic. They are creative, quick to action, talkative and very social and they dislike routine. On the negative side, people with vata dominant can be indecisive, scattered, flighty and nervous. An Ayurvedic practitioner would most likely recommend grounding techniques, a regular sleep-eat schedule and perhaps walking meditation.

Healing recommendations for vatas:

➤ Avoid extreme cold, dress appropriately for temperature

➤ Practice stress management

➤ Avoid cold, frozen or raw foods; eat warm spicy foods

➤ Keep a regular routine

➤ Get plenty of rest

Pitta, the fire dosha: They generally have a medium build, pale skin that sunburns easily. They have an intense appetite, gain and lose weight easily and dislike heat and humidity. By temperament, they are leaders: bright, intelligent, arrogant, driven, direct, witty, competitive and intense.

Unbalanced pitta results in rash decisions and self-destructive behavior. Physically, this can manifest as skin conditions like rashes, eczema and acne, inflammation and digestive issues. It can also result in hormonal and metabolic imbalances.

Healing recommendations for pittas:

➤ Eat cooler foods lie those found in a Mediterranean diet

➤ Cooling, calming activities like swimming

➤ Sufficient relaxation, meditation

➤ At least seven hours of sleep a night

Kapha, the earth dosha: People with dominant kapha are broad, strong, athletic and curvy. They are generally calm, steady, grounded, stubborn and slow learners with long memories. Eating is their great passion, so they tend to have a lifelong battle with their weight. Kaphas don't like cool, damp climates. They like leisurely activity and deeply value peace and inner tranquility.

They like routine. Physically, they are susceptible to overweight and food cravings, especially for sweets and fatty foods. They are susceptible to respiratory and bronchial infections and tend to sleep too much, especially during the day.

Unbalanced Kapha leads to lack of motivation, emotional withdrawal, stubbornness and unwillingness to change, even when change is necessary.

Healing recommendations for kaphas:

➢ Regular exercise routine

➢ Active lifestyle with lots of social interaction

➢ Diet rich in low fat, spicy foods

➢ Occasional fasting

➢ Avoid napping

This is just the barest description of Ayurveda. We strongly recommend that you take a deeper dive into this traditional form of medicine that has served the people of India for millennia and continues to serve them to this day.

Traditional Chinese Medicine

This ancient Chinese system of medicine focuses on psychological and/or physical approaches, such as acupuncture, a specific type of Chinese massage, tai chi, nutritional approaches and herbal products to address health problems.

Known to be 3,500 years older than Western conventional medicine, TCM revers the Daoist belief that the human body is a miniature version of the universe. A key element of TCM is that a vital energy called Qi flows through the body and performs multiple functions to maintain health. TCM practitioners believe that chronic pain results from blockage or imbalance of Qi, and that their role is to correct or balance its flow.

Opposing or balancing forces called Yin and Yang are also important element of TCM. Practitioners seek to balance the polarity of those forces often referred to as feminine (yin) and masculine (yang).

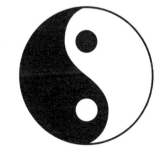

TCM practitioners use a variety of diagnostic techniques, including looking at the tongue and testing pulses in several parts of the body.

While TCM is best known for pain relief for migraine and for surgeries performed under acupuncture anesthesia with no pain for the patient, it has also been documented to enhance the immune system and prevent disease as well as treating anxiety, depression, chronic pain, chemical dependency, women's health, PMS and menopause, digestive disorders, musculoskeletal pain and much more.

Traditional Chinese herbal medicines come in the form of raw herbs, powdered extractions, tinctures, pills, capsules and essential oils. They can be derived from any part of the plant including the rhizome, roots, seeds or flowers. Minerals and animal products are sometimes included in the herbal formulations.

Basic elements of TCM

Acupuncture usually involves inserting thin needles through the skin to stimulate specific points called meridians to restore balance and healing.

According to the National Institutes of Health (NIH), "Studies suggest that acupuncture stimulates the release of the body's natural painkillers and affects areas in the brain involved in processing pain; however, some trials suggest that real acupuncture and sham acupuncture (similar to real acupuncture, except that needles are not actually inserted into the skin) are equally effective, indicating a placebo effect.

"Results from a number of studies, however, suggest real acupuncture may help ease types of pain that are often chronic, such as low-back pain, neck pain, osteoarthritis/knee pain, and carpal tunnel syndrome. It also may help reduce the frequency of tension headaches and prevent migraine headaches," the NIH concludes.

Tai Chi

Tai chi is characterized by gentle movements, mental focus, breathing, postures and relaxation that has many parallels to the Indian practice of yoga. Practicing tai chi has been scientifically validated to improve balance and stability in older people and those with Parkinson's disease, reduce pain from knee osteoarthritis, help people cope with fibromyalgia and back pain, and promote quality of life and improve mood in people with heart failure.

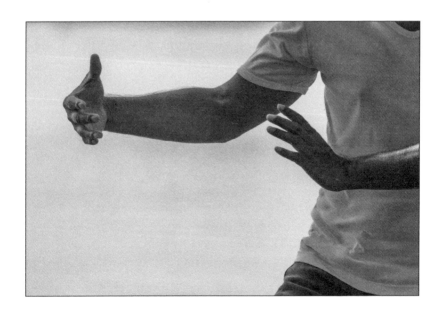

Chinese Herbal Products

Chinese herbal products have been studied for many medical problems, including stroke, heart disease, mental disorders, and respiratory diseases (such as bronchitis and the common cold), and a national survey showed that about one in five Americans use them.

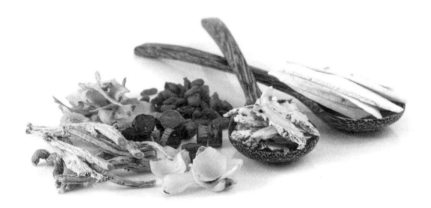

Do your homework if you're considering using botanicals since many have been shown to contain less than the listed amount of their ingredients and some even contain toxic materials and pharmaceuticals that should only be available by prescription and under a doctor's supervision.

Look for a reputable brand with products that have undergone extensive testing, ideally by a third-party lab, and are sourced from high quality ingredients.

How to choose the best botanical for you:

1. Read the ingredients. Labels should always include the botanical name of plants used, the plant parts used and the amount standardized in each dose.

2. The recommended dosage and frequency.

3. A listing of other ingredients that might be included, including gluten.

4. Consider the cost. Cheapest is usually not the best.

5. Look for a label certifying "non-GMO" and laboratory tested for purity and quality.

Practitioners

Most states and the District of Columbia have laws regulating acupuncture practice, and most states require certification from the National Certification Commission for Acupuncture and Oriental Medicine.

Resources

NIH Fact Sheets

Acupuncture:
https://www.nccih.nih.gov/health/acupuncture-what-you-need-to-know

Tai Chi:
https://www.nccih.nih.gov/health/tai-chi-what-you-need-to-know

CHAPTER 9

Other Forms of Alternative Medicine

This chapter could actually be an encyclopedia (anybody remember those?), but we'd like to give you a basic idea of the many forms of alternative medicine that are scientifically validated to have a measurable impact on your wellbeing.

This is far from a full listing. Please feel free to explore further on your own beyond these modalities and those mentioned in the previous chapters.

As we've mentioned, alternative medicine differs from conventional medicine's approach of a single target when treating disease. Alternative medicine embraces the whole human organism: body, mind and spirit. Some therapies target one element of this triad with the intent of unlocking blockages in the other two. Others embrace two or even all three.

BODY

Massage

Deep tissue (sometimes called myofascial) and neuromuscular massage are both validated to work against chronic pain in different ways. Both involve deep and sometimes painful release work.

Deep tissue massage focuses on painful areas and stiff muscles, tendons and tissues deep within your skin. Neuromuscular

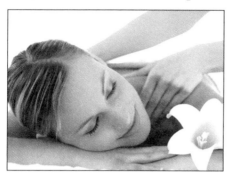

massage focuses on releasing nerves. Both trigger a pressure, release and relaxation response in the affected areas.

Several studies have validated both forms of massage, especially to relieve chronic pain, postural misalignments, migraines and lymphedema in breast cancer patients. Frequently both therapies are used in the same session.

Bodywork

While it can include various types of massage, bodywork can include yoga, tai chi, acupressure and more. As mentioned in earlier chapters, both yoga and tai chi have been well studied for their benefits in managing stress, combatting depression, promoting weight loss (especially targeting dangerous abdominal fat), improving quality sleep, maintaining flexibility, improving

cognitive ability in the elderly and improving balance and much more.

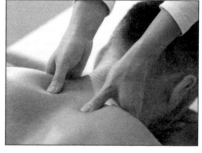

In addition, both yoga and tai chi traditionally incorporate breath work and meditation that can expand their effectiveness.

Acupressure is similar to acupuncture without the needles. Practitioners use fingers or devices to press on the meridian points, giving similar results, helping relieve pain and enhancing the circulation of *qi, chi* or *prana* energy for overall healing.

Diet and Fasting

A natural diet based on unprocessed foods, healthy fats, organic foods whenever possible and natural body recovery time between meals is a cornerstone of a healthy body.

Voluminous research shows that a diet high in fresh fruits and vegetables, healthy fats, whole grains and moderate consumption of meat and fish is best for almost everyone.

Dr. Goel is of the strong conviction that most of us consume far too many calories, regardless of where those calories are coming from.

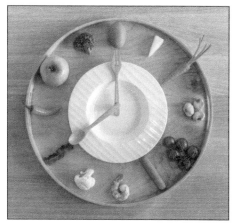

The ancient practice of fasting generally means abstaining for most or all food and drink (except water) for a set period of time, usually 24–72 hours, sometimes longer. Resting the digestive system for a few hours or a few days has been scientifically proven to have a host of health benefits, including reducing inflammation, which is at the core of many chronic health issues.

Fasting has been associated with a wide array of potential health benefits, including weight loss, cancer prevention and improved blood sugar control, heart health and brain function.

Intermittent fasting is a more recent practice in which eating is concentrated within a specific number of hours a day or days a week. Most frequently, people practicing intermittent fasting eat in an 8-hour window and fasting 16 hours) has recently been touted as a weight loss tool. While the research is mixed, some studies confirm that fasting bring the body into a state called ketosis, which assists in weight loss by burning fat for energy.

Supplements

It should go without saying that supplements that target specific health issues and promote overall wellness are a core part of

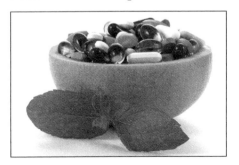

any healing plan. They are so important that we've devoted the entire next chapter to the use of supplements, why they are important for virtually everyone and how to choose the right ones.

MIND

It's hard to separate mind and spirit sometimes, but we'll give it a try here. Even standard or conventional medicine recognizes the power of the connection between mind and body. Studies have found that people heal better if they have good emotional and mental health.

Guided imagery

This very effective relaxation tool is induced by a voice (a coach or a recording) leading you to a variety of soothing images. You will probably be asked to visualize a favorite scene in nature and you'll be asked to engage all of your senses to bring yourself of that

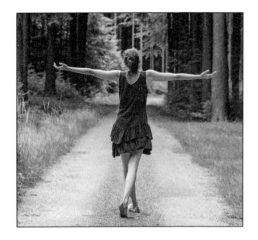

place, which results in a state of deep relaxation. For example, if your peaceful place is in a forest, you might be asked to see the deep, cool shade of the forest, smell the pine needles, hear the wind in the trees and feel the gentle breeze on your skin.

After an initial session, you may be able to induce the guided imagery on your own.

Guided imagery if most often used to create a feeling of general wellbeing. It has been proven effective in relieving post-operative pain in children, reducing pain in patients with advanced cancer and helping improve gait in people who have had strokes.

Progressive muscle relaxation

This technique involves slowly tensing and relaxing muscle groups. It has been proven to reduce stress and anxiety, improve sleep, reduce chronic pain and even improve breathing in people with COPD (Chronic Obstructive Pulmonary Disease). It has generally been validated to have similar benefits as guided imagery.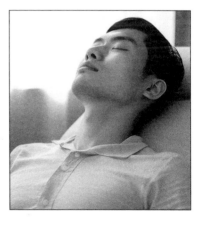

It's simple to practice and once you've been led through a session (there are multiple online resources), you can reproduce the technique on your own.

Hypnotherapy

This form of deep relaxation and focused concentration is administered by a trained and certified hypnotherapist who guides subjects into state of deep relaxation using verbal cues, repetitive instructions and imagery. This genuine psychological therapy

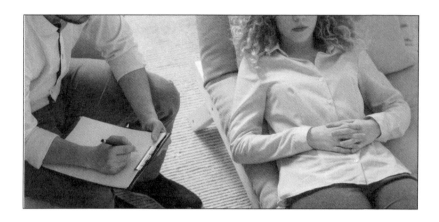

can create an open mind to treatment suggestions. It is frequently used to help stop smoking, for example, with measurable success.

Hypnotherapy has also been proven effective in treating insomnia, irritable bowel syndrome, menopausal symptoms, bladder incontinence and post-operative pain.

Biofeedback

This mind-body technique is used to help subjects control some body functions, such as heart rate, breathing patterns and muscle responses. During biofeedback, you're connected to electrical pads that help you get information about your body. Biofeedback is often combined with mindfulness-based meditation. Partic-

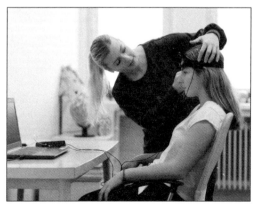

ipants in a Dutch study found long lasting beneficial effects from biofeedback, including reduced stress, anxiety and depressive symptoms, improved psychological well-being and sleep quality.

SPIRIT

Spiritually based therapies were at the core of our ancestors' medical knowledge. Some therapies that seemed mystical at the time are now better understood by modern science. They are very effective today.

Meditation

This umbrella term includes many practices, all of which involve focusing the mind focus on a particular object, thought or activity, most commonly on the breath in a popular form called mindfulness meditation. It's an element of many religions although it is not specifically a religious practice, meditation is intended to help practitioners achieve a mentally clear and emotionally calm and stable state.

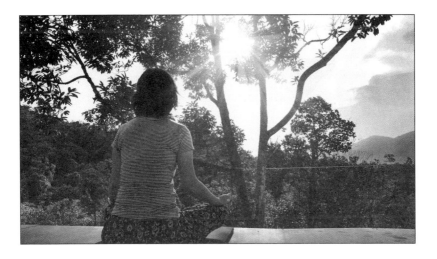

Meditation has become increasingly popular in the United States with approximately 14% of adults regularly practicing some form, a threefold increase over the past five years.

It has been deeply studied with overwhelmingly positive results. In addition to the generally recognized effects of meditation in relieving stress, anxiety and depression, it has been scientifically validated to improve brain, sleep and immune function, reduce blood pressure and relieve chronic pain. Some of the most exciting studies show that meditation can improve memory, including in people with dementia and help break addictions to alcohol and drugs.

Meditation is incredibly easily accessible. It can be practiced by anyone, anywhere.

Supplements: Proof They Work

Reasons why food isn't enough

"I eat a healthy diet. Most of my food is organic and unprocessed. So why do I need supplements?" you are probably asking.

That's a good question. And there are very good answers.

First: It's extremely difficult to get all our nutrition from food. That sounds counter intuitive and outrageous, we know.

Today's combination of depleted soil and poor nutrient quality of what we grow, thanks to the greedy food industry, makes it close to impossible to get all the nutrients we need from food.

Soil depletion

Modern agricultural methods have stripped our soil of its nutrients, making our food less nutritious, less sustaining. Excessively intense cultivation and poor soil management have resulted in higher yields and less nutrition.

Based on data on 43 fruits and vegetables from the U.S. Department of Agriculture studied from 1950 to 1999, researchers at the University of Texas at Austin found "reliable declines" in the amount of protein, calcium, phosphorus, iron, riboflavin (vitamin B2) and vitamin C. The study attributes this declining nutritional content to the preponderance of agricultural practices designed to improve traits (size, growth rate, pest resistance) other than nutrition. We can only assume that the nutrient decline has worsened in the past 24 years since the study was concluded.

So, is the carrot you are eating today as nutritious as the one you might have eaten in 1970 or 1950?

No, says *Scientific American*. Worse yet, "Each successive generation of fast-growing, pest-resistant carrot is truly less good for you than the one before."

In addition, there have likely been declines in other key nutrients, too, researchers said, including magnesium, zinc and vitamins B-6 and E, but they were not studied in 1950.

"A similar study of British nutrient data from 1930 to 1980, published in the *British Food Journal*, found that in 20 vegetables the average calcium content had declined 19 percent; iron 22

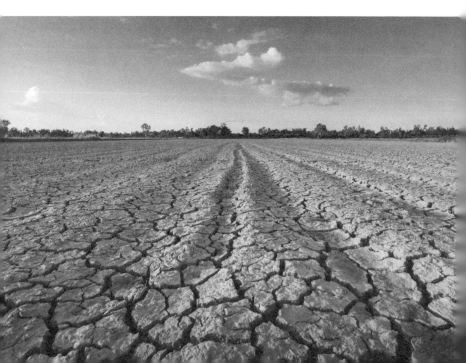

percent; and potassium 14 percent. Yet another study concluded that one would have to eat eight oranges today to derive the same amount of Vitamin A as our grandparents would have gotten from one," says the 2011 *Scientific American* article.

A 2015 study from the University of California at Berkeley warned that soil depletion poses a "huge risk to global food security over the next century."

They concluded, "...past and future human activities will play a major role in human prosperity and survival."

It probably goes without saying that nutritionally depleted food sources result in even worse nutrition based on the Standard American Diet of highly processed and nutritionally void convenience foods with excessive amounts of saturated fats, and we are quite literally starving ourselves of the nutrients we need while becoming fatter and fatter. It's a recipe for a global health disaster.

What to do?

This is serious, friends. Yes, we can and should lobby the food industry to change agricultural practices. We can and should ask our legislators to put restrictions on farming techniques and the use of pesticides and herbicides in place, but it may be too late.

Definitely don't stop eating fruits and vegetables. They are still "extraordinarily rich in nutrients and beneficial phytochemicals," say the authors of the University of Texas study.

Whenever possible, buy locally from organic growers, but supplementation is the answer for virtually everyone now.

It should go without saying that supplements that target specific health issues and promote overall wellness are a core part of any healing plan. They are so important that we've devoted this entire section to discussing the use of some specific supplements that we have studied extensively, why they are important for virtually everyone and how to choose the right ones.

CHAPTER 10

The Right Supplements

onfused? That's not surprising! Ready to roll? That's not surprising, either.

The huge range of supplements available would confuse anyone. In this chapter, we're going to present to you abbreviated information on the supplements with which we are the most familiar, some of which Dr. Goel has studied extensively.

While they have all been found to be effective and safe to prevent and treat a wide range of diseases, we like to think of some of them as today's botanical daily regimen for healthy and longevity.

In the next chapter, we'll give you some tools to help you decide which ones to buy and how much to take.

So, without further fanfare, here are the pieces of the health puzzle that we think everyone should be taking every day:

Curcumin (*Curcuma longa*)

This powerhouse botanical comes from the rhizome (root bulb) of the plant that produces the Indian spice, curry. It is at the top of our list of supplements to be taken daily for its huge array of health benefits.

> Curcumin has shown positive effects in treating every single disease for which it has been studied.

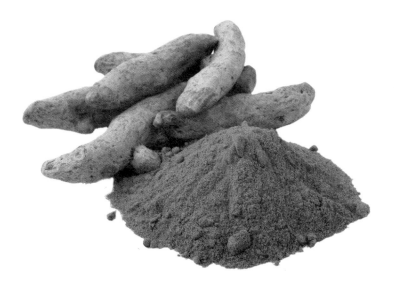

There are more than 21,000 studies on the impressive range of benefits curcumin can provide.

Curcumin is among the best studied of all botanicals. Research confirms that curcumin and its active ingredients, called curcuminoids, are safe and effective against:

> Heart disease, especially high blood pressure and high blood fats and cholesterol;

> Metabolic syndrome, the combination of high blood pressure, high cholesterol, high blood sugar and excess weight around the waist that dramatically increases the risk of heart attack and stroke;

> Anxiety and depression that affects more than 21 million American adults, including half of those between the ages of 18 and 24;

> Alzheimer's disease by combatting the beta amyloid plaques that cause brain deterioration and memory loss;

> Joint pain and arthritis.

More than 7,000 studies have been published on curcumin's anti-cancer activity alone. Dr. Goel has personally conducted more than 30 published studies that prove curcumin fights and prevents cancer through at least five pathways, unlike any other botanical or pharmaceutical known to science.

Note: Many forms of curcumin are poorly absorbed. Look for a product that is confirmed to be absorbable. Despite popular opinion, the addition of piperine (black pepper) alone is not sufficient to ensure your body can actually use the curcumin you are taking.

Also, turmeric is the spice that comes from the same plant as curcumin. Curcumin is medicinal. You won't get the benefits of curcumin by taking turmeric.

French Grape Seed Extract (*Vitis vinifera*) (FGSE)

We like to think of FGSE as Mother Nature's multi-tasker. The active ingredients, called oligomeric proanthocyanidins, affect virtually every metabolic function in the human body.

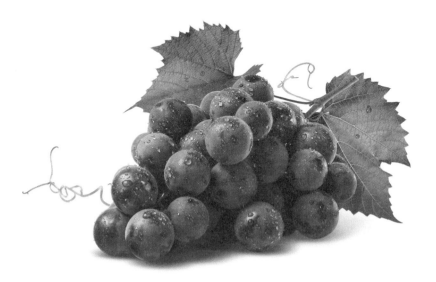

FGSE is a high-powered botanical rich in anti-inflammatory and antioxidant compounds. That makes it an impressive weapon to prevent and fight common diseases and health challenges.

Lab studies show that the active ingredients in FGSE are much more effective than vitamin C and vitamin E and virtually any type of food in neutralizing those health destroying free radical oxygen molecules.

The antioxidant levels in French grape seed extract are so high they are quite literally off the scale. The ORAC (oxygen radical absorbance capacity) value of FGSE is so high it is difficult even for modern equipment to accurately measure it. ORAC values are a measure of the free-radical fighting capabilities of a particular food.

Among its most researched anti-inflammatory and antioxidant properties are:

➤ Reverses heart disease by lowering blood pressure, cholesterol and blood fats;

➤ Prevents and treats cancer in several ways, including by stopping the spread of cancerous cells (metastasis) and preventing the return of cancers after remission;

➤ Improves blood sugar regulation in Type 2 diabetes, thereby offering protection against its dire side effects, including heart disease, stroke, kidney disease, amputations, blindness and more;

➤ Assists in weight loss and weight maintenance;

➤ Protects the brain against beta amyloid plaque, preventing and perhaps reversing Alzheimer's disease;

➤ Helps circumvent faulty brain "circuitry" to create new information pathways if older ones break down;

➤ Speeds wound healing;

> Stops infections caused by at least 10 different bacteria, including MRSA, an antibiotic resistant infection often found in hospital settings, which can be fatal;

> Increases lifespan in lab animals.

We're learning more about French grape seed extract's impressive powers against disease and its ability to promote a long, healthy life nearly every day, so a compendium of its benefits will always fall short. For now, let's just l eave it that we think *everyone* should take FGSE every day. There's no downside and uncountable upsides.

Andrographis (*Andrographis paniculata*)

Little known outside of Asia, andrographis has been widely used in the Ayurvedic medical tradition. Its value has been validated by extensive Western research.

Andrographis is also often called "The King of Bitters," meaning it tastes extremely bitter. That's why you'd probably want to take it in capsules as it's most commonly found. In herbal traditions around the world, bitter herbs usually have cleansing

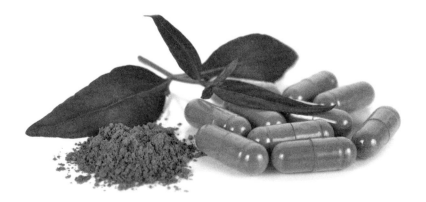

and temperature-regulating effects and improve circulation, benefit the nervous system and cool the body's inflammatory response.

Andrographolides, the active ingredients in andrographis, are a rare group of diterpenoid lactones, which have strong proven antimicrobial, anti-inflammatory and antioxidant effects. Modern science confirms that andrographis is also a rich source of other nutrients, including well-researched antioxidant flavonoids and polyphenols, giving it a broad range of health benefits.

Known as an adaptogen, a compound that helps return your body to balance, andrographis actually works like a stress vaccine to activate the body's defense system and metabolic rate to reverse the negative effects of stress and restore the body to balance and health.

Perhaps the greatest value of andrographis is its ability to enhance immune function. Not only does andrographis bring about balance in the body, it's inarguably your body's most powerful ally against the onslaught of pathogenic challenges launched at it every day. It's proven effective against virtually all types of infections: viral, bacterial, parasitic and fungal.

If your immune system is not functioning properly by overreacting or underreacting to challenges like viral infections, andrographis supports the correct immune response.

It's an additional powerful weapon against cancer. Probably the most impressive overview of the pertinent research comes from an international consortium of 19 scientists that confirmed andrographis' anticancer effects "on almost all types of cell lines" on at least five different ways. That's makes andrographis one our best defenses against cancer.

Andrographis' other most confirmed effects:

➢ Antiviral, especially against several strains of influenza, including COVID-19 and HIV;

➤ Antibacterial, including against *Staphylococcus aureus*. Lyme disease, MRSA and more;

➤ Control and reverse non-alcoholic fatty liver disease;

➤ Enhance liver function and even revive it when there has been a liver disease, often used as a treatment for all forms of hepatitis.

As you can see form its unique properties, andrographis is another important tool in your disease fighting arsenal.

If that's not enough to convince you, andrographis has also been proven to work synergistically with other botanicals (including curcumin) to enhance the disease fighting properties of both.

Berberine (*Berberis vulgaris*)

Dr. Goel has conducted several studies on the alkaloid compound berberine and he's an enthusiastic supporter of this little-known botanical for several reasons.

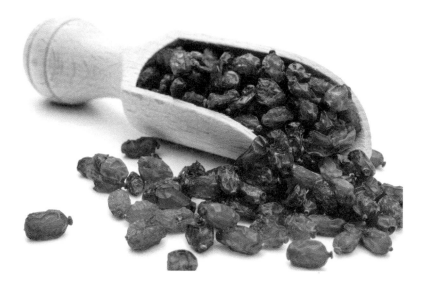

One of the most impressive and unique properties of berberine is its ability to help lengthen telomeres. These caps at the ends of DNA strands become frayed or shortened as we age, so cells die. When this happens, we are more susceptible to the diseases of aging and our lives are shortened. Telomeres are known as the primary indicators of aging and predictors of mortality in humans.

A healthy lifestyle, and especially a healthy diet, have been scientifically proven to prevent telomeres from shortening. That's where berberine comes in, since it is also validated as a way to protect those end caps, thereby reducing the risk of disease and promoting a long, healthy life.

Telomere protection is also a key factor in overcoming all types of cancers. Dr. Goel's research shows berberine has the rare ability to strengthen the body's defenses against cancer especially overcoming resistance to the chemotherapy agent, gemcitabine, not only in colorectal cancers, but also in often deadly pancreatic cancers.

Berberine has been proven effective in preventing metabolic syndrome, which is a cluster of disease factors including high blood pressure, elevated cholesterol, high triglycerides, high blood sugar and obesity that vastly increases the risk of diabetes and heart disease.

Berberine is also validated to:

➤ Promote weight loss

➤ Control blood sugars;

➤ Reverse congestive heart failure;

➤ Promote weight loss, especially reducing belly fat;

➤ Reverse fatty liver disease, primarily caused by excess belly fat;

➤ Normalize blood fats and cholesterol, reducing the risk of heart attacks and strokes.

➤ Enhance blood sugar control;

➤ Activate AMPK, a fat-burning enzyme that helps cells re-energize when their fuel sources are low and prevents wild cell division like we find in cancer;

Red Ginseng (*Panax ginseng*)

This effective treatment for cancer, diabetes, erectile dysfunction and menopausal symptoms has been prized as an adaptogen in Traditional Chinese Medicine.

Its active ginsenosides, also known as steroid-like saponins, are responsible for many of the herb's healing qualities. Some of the most important fight inflammation, neutralize disease-causing free radicals and protect nerve cells that attack cancer in a variety of ways. Other ginsenosides in red ginseng address the underlying causes of Alzheimer's disease and dozens more disease conditions.

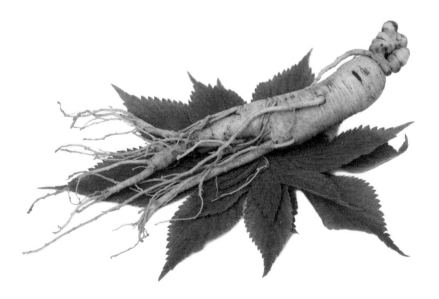

These major ginsenosides can be converted into rare ginsenosides by microorganisms in the digestive tract, making them potent healing agents.

Red ginseng's confirmed properties:

➤ Immune enhancement

➤ Anti-tumor

➤ Relieves mental and physical fatigue (tonic and energizer)

➤ Treatment for Chronic Fatigue Syndrome and fibromyalgia

➤ Relieves chronic pain

➤ Calmative by reducing cortisol production for stress relief

➤ Antidepressant

➤ Improves brain function, mental clarity and memory, decreases age-related cognitive decline and the risk of cerebral ischemia

Greek Mountain Tea (*Sideritis scardica*) (GMT)

GMT's considerable healing properties are attributed to anti-inflammatory aromatic essential oils and antioxidant-rich polyphenols and flavonoids.

In today's science, Alzheimer's disease researchers are focusing research on GMT as a potential treatment and preventive for various forms of dementia.

Modern scientific research confirms GMT can:

➤ Combat Alzheimer's disease and cognitive decline;

➤ Lower blood pressure, reducing the risk of heart attacks and strokes;

➤ Improve digestive health;

➤ Increase bone density;

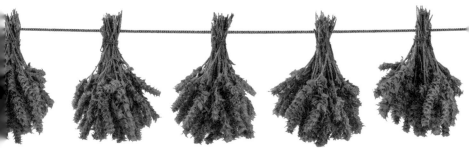

➤ Enhance immune function and prevent colds and flu;

➤ Reduce anxiety and depression;

➤ Reduce insulin resistance and the risk of type 2 diabetes;

➤ Promote weight loss;

➤ Relieve joint pain.

While the ancient Greeks typically consumed GMT as a brewed tea, today's science gives us the same benefits in a convenient capsule.

We recommend adding *Bacopa monnieri* to your GMT for an additional stress buster.

Finally...

Dr. Goel's research has confirmed that some of these botanicals work synergistically, meaning when you take two or more of them together, they enhance one another's healing power.

Have you noticed a pattern here? All of the botanicals in this chapter are powerhouse anti-inflammatories and antioxidants, making them the most effective weapons against chronic diseases of all sorts.

That's why we enthusiastically recommend them all as your personalized health insurance policy.

Dosage Recommendations

➤ Curcumin with proven bioavailability with turmeric essential oil: 750 mg 2–3 softgel capsules daily for those who have been diagnosed with cancer

➤ Andrographis: 400 mg standardized at 20% yielding 80 mg of andrographolides, 400 mg 2–3 times daily

➤ French grape seed extract: tannin free, 400 mg soft-gel capsules, 2–3 daily

➤ Berberine with gamma-cyclodextrin: 250–500 mg daily

➤ Red ginseng with gamma-cyclodextrin: 100 mg chewable tablet daily

➤ Greek Mountain Tea: 450 mg daily plus 200 mg *Bacopa monnieri*

If you want to take a deeper look at these supplements and get detailed references, please investigate through these books:

Beat Cancer Naturally Now! The Five Most Powerful Natural Alternatives to Prevent and Treat Cancer. Ajay Goel, Ph.D., AGAF and Terry Lemerond. TTN Publishing, 2023.

Greek Mountain Tea: The Key to Mental Clarity and More. Terry Lemerond. TTN Publishing, 2023.

Discover Andrographis. Alex Panossian, Ph.D., Dr. Sci and Terry Lemerond, TTN Publishing 2023.

French Grape Seed Extract: Prevent and Reverse Cancer, Heart Disease, Diabetes, Alzheimer's and More. Ajay Goel, M.S., Ph.D and Terry Lemerond. TTN Publishing, 2023.

Red Ginseng: The Asian Heal All Herb. Jacob Teitelbaum. M.D. and Terry Lemerond. TTN Publishing. 2022.

CHAPTER 11

How to Choose
the Right Supplements

We're the first to agree with you that there are overwhelming numbers of products on the market, and it can be extremely difficult to choose those that will be effective and not break your budget.

How can you navigate those choppy waters?

Here's what we've both discovered in our combined decades of research on natural products:

➤ The cheapest product is usually not the best.

➤ Your supplement should be GMO free.

➤ Look for products manufactured in a cGMP (current good manufacturing practices) compliant facility.

➤ The label should reveal if the product contains sugar, salt, yeast, wheat, gluten, corn, soy, dairy products, artificial coloring, artificial flavoring or preservatives.

Botanicals are made up of hundreds of molecules that work on multiple pathways in the body at multiple levels of those pathways, all simultaneously. Botanicals are like having a pharmacy in a bottle without the fear of side effects. Pharmaceuticals, especially those that target cancer in various ways, are limited to what they can accomplish since they are composed of one molecule targeting one pathway in the body, thereby throwing many other pathways out of balance, and the benefits are limited as well.

Bioavailability

The key to results is not how many milligrams of supplements or nutrients you take orally, but how many milligrams your body can absorb from the intestines into the blood. Only the amount you absorb can have a biological effect on your health. In the past, researchers have thought curcumin and berberine were difficult to absorb, but new research shows that certain types of processing and additions to the ingredients make them super absorbable and super effective.

In our experience, these natural ingredients can have impressive long-term benefits. Extensive research confirms those benefits. Botanicals are free from the side effects and complications caused by pharmaceuticals. More and more physicians are beginning to see that the side effects of drugs often outweigh their benefits.

Patients always ask us what brands we recommend. That's such an important question because there are so many brands on the market. Some are basically worthless, while there are other high-quality brands you can always depend on. We recommend visiting your local health food store for help identifying products of the highest and most consistent quality in the industry, and which are sustainably produced and standardized.

Curcumin

Curcumin doesn't work like an aspirin. You can't swallow it with a glass of water and expect it to take care of the problem. That means it *must* work in another way. What we know for sure is that it *does* work!

Curcumin is fat soluble. When it is taken by mouth, curcumin is detectable in the brain, which may in part explain its effectiveness in preventing and treating brain diseases.

The curcumin Dr. Goel uses in his research is curcumin rhizome blended with essential oils from turmeric based on the centuries-old Ayurveda system, so the product is all natural. It has been shown to have 7 to 10 times higher bioavailability and research shows it is retained longer in the circulatory system than standard curcumin. There are curcumin products that claim higher bioavailability, but their fatty coating is synthetic. Additionally, it is very important to have label information confirming that turmeric essential oil contains turmerones, which are themselves anticancer and have been shown to boost the activity of curcumin.

One study shows that this curcumin has a double peak action. It shows up in the bloodstream of human subjects within an hour and drops for a short period of time, then rises again 4.5 hours later and remains detectable in the blood after eight hours. That means not only is it absorbed, it remains in the system much longer than other curcumin supplements, which typically dissipate within a little more than 2 hours.

This formulation is clearly superior because it is easily absorbed and contains compounds (turmerones) that boost curcumin's effectiveness.

Curcumin is often combined with boswellia (also known as frankincense), for increased anti-inflammatory effects.

French Grape Seed Extract

Bioavailability is essential to the efficacy of any treatment. The best French grape seed extract product should be tannin-free, since tannins inhibit absorption. Small molecular structure is also important to bioavailability.

In our opinion, the best FGSE product is a formulation that has >99% polyphenols and >80% OPCs.

This unique extract is never adulterated and is standardized for only small size OPCs to better ensure absorption. You won't go wrong if you use this formulation.

Recommended dosage is 400 mg daily, and up to 1,200 mg daily for people with active cancers. There have been no significant documented side effects.

Andrographis

You'll get the best results with 400 mg of andrographis standardized at 20% andrographolides 1–3 times daily.

Some people choose to take andrographis on a temporary basis for 7 to 10 days to treat colds or flu or other acute infections. Others take it for years on end to treat serious health issues such as cancer or heart disease, or cognitive dysfunction with no apparent negative effects. You can safely take 1 to 4 times the recommended dosages if you have serious health conditions like these.

Andrographis has long been associated with liver health. Its antiviral properties make it effective against hepatitis C. It can arrest fibrosis, a condition that can lead to dangerous cirrhosis. Andrographis has also been shown to completely eradicate 80% of cases of infectious hepatitis. Recent research confirms that it can treat and even reverse non-alcoholic fatty liver disease.

The most frequently reported side effect was a mild skin rash that disappeared as soon as people stopped taking the herb.

Anaphylaxis, a severe and life-threatening allergic reaction, has been reported in a handful of people taking andrographis in very high dosages, over 5 grams daily.

Red Ginseng

Red Ginseng is also known as Asian or Korean red ginseng.

To ensure you're getting a clean *Panax ginseng* product, check the front label for the words "whole root," "full spectrum," and "solvent-free." You want a supplement that is GMO-free and hasn't been irradiated or been adulterated in any way.

The best product is processed using traditional Korean steam cooking and drying methods that make it safe, clean and effective. Look for a product that is grown hydroponically without any toxic chemicals. The clean production process concentrates rare ginsenosides, making it by far the most effective red ginseng formulation available.

Greek Mountain Tea

We prefer Greek mountain tea processed, tested and standardized into capsules for consistent levels of polyphenols. This is the only way we know of to be certain you are getting a clean product that will do what you need it to do, since Greek mountain tea is usually wildcrafted without a supply chain that ensures safety.

Look for a product that is lab tested for purity and quality and contains 500 mg of Greek mountain tea per capsule with a recommended dosage of one or two a day, depending on whether you are taking it for preventive purposes or as a treatment, when the higher dose would be advisable. All you need is one or two capsules daily.

Greek Mountain Tea is sometimes combined with *Bacopa monnieri* for additional stress relief.

The capsules are reassurance of getting exactly what is needed every single day. It's much more convenient, especially if you travel often, as we do.

Berberine

Berberine is notoriously difficult for the human body to absorb. In the past, extremely large doses were necessary to get the desired results, especially in regulating metabolic syndrome. But recent research shows that gamma cyclodextrin, an oligosaccharide (plant-based ingredient) improves the absorption of certain fat-soluble nutrients up to eight-fold. It also speeds up the body's response to berberine and other botanicals.

Look for a root and bark extract from *Berberis aristata*, also known as Indian Barberry (*Berberis aristata*) with 500 mg of berberine, the amount found effective in clinical studies.

We recommend up to three capsules daily.

CHAPTER 12

Doc to Doc

Most authors are protective of their work and prohibit copying and distributing book contents unless they are sold or pay a fee.

This section of this book is very different. This information is so important that we want to see it distributed far and wide. At least as far as this chapter goes, we are unconcerned about copyright.

We also know that doctors and other healthcare practitioners are very busy. They are very unlikely to read an entire book, even though, like this book, it may contain some information that could save the lives or help improve the quality of life of their patients. We understand that doctors are frequently skeptical about natural formulations and, if they haven't conducted their own research investigations on a subject, they are inclined to steer their patients away from them, even though these formulations might be lifesaving.

We've created this short chapter, a synopsis of the most important elements of this book. We encourage you to copy it freely. Give it to your doctor or other healthcare practitioner and encourage them to spend 10 minutes reading and digesting these few pages.

Dear Doctor,

Your patient has given you a copy of this chapter with my blessings and permission. My publisher and I have given it to the public domain so that the vital information it contains on the value of curcumin, other significant botanicals in prevention and treatment of a wide range of cancers can be broadly circulated.

In this book, I am specifically examining varying practices generally termed "alternative" medicine.

I have spent more than 20 years researching the preventive and treatment properties of botanicals, primarily for cancer prevention and treatment, in my previous tenure at Baylor University and my current tenure at the City of Hope.

I've published more than 400 studies on various aspects of health and cancer, including numerous studies emphasizing the health benefits of complementary and alternative medicine and treatments based on Traditional Chinese Medicine and Ayurvedic tradition.

I urge you to take a few minutes to read this section and consider how alternative, holistic, integrative, complementary, functional or precision medicine—whatever you call it—will benefit your patients.

—Ajay Goel, Ph.D., M.S., City of Hope Professor and Chair,
Department of Molecular Diagnostics and Experimental Therapeutics;
Associate Director of Basic Science, Comprehensive Cancer Center
(formerly Baylor University's Center for Gastrointestinal Research and
the Center for Epigenetics, Cancer Prevention and Cancer Genomics)

Dear Healthcare Professional,

So, what is alternative medicine? It's known by many names, most based on ancient knowledge that is now validated by modern science. I'm using "alternative" medicine as a general term to delineate therapies outside the realm of conventional medicine that can work with modern therapies or in addition to these therapies to bring about healing.

In the past, you may have dismissed alternative therapies out of hand as "kooky," or "scientifically unsound." I'm the first to agree that there have been some "kooky" ideas out there.

However, I urge you to take a few minutes for self-education to learn more about therapies that are extensively studied, scientifically validated and safe and efficacious.

Yes, modern science does validate the efficacy and safety of many "alternative therapies," including yoga, meditation, massage therapy, nutritional awareness, lifestyle changes, botanical and mineral supplementation.

As a cancer researcher, I'll focus on the use of botanicals in this chapter.

For more than 20 years, we have known that American soils are depleted and producing crops that are nutritionally diminished to the point where, in my opinion, it is nearly impossible for the average person to glean essential nutrients from fruits and vegetables for disease prevention, much less disease treatment.

In this book, I've recommended a handful of basic supplements that can help overcome these systemic deficiencies for disease prevention and treatment. Since I'm a cancer researcher and I've personally engaged in extensive research of many of them, I can attest that all are validated for safety and efficacy by peer-reviewed studies.

You will note that virtually all of my recommended botanicals are potent anti-inflammatory and antioxidant agents. This is essential to their broad efficacy in preventing and treating numerous disease conditions, primarily the chronic diseases of aging.

Curcumin (*Curcuma longa*): More than 7,000 studies have been published on curcumin's anti-cancer activity alone. Benefits have been documented dating back to 1983, but the vast majority have been published in the past 20 years. I've personally conducted more than 30 such studies. I can personally affirm curcumin's value in preventing carcinogenesis, angiogenesis, apoptosis, metastasis, chemoprotection, chemo-enhancement and metastasis through cancer stem cells through a broad range of pathways, unlike any pharmaceutical known to science.

In addition, curcumin and its active ingredients, curcuminoids, are well-researched and validated to prevent and treat:

➢ Hyperlipidemia

➢ Metabolic syndrome

➢ Anxiety and depression

➢ Alzheimer's disease by increasing levels of BDNF

Curcumin has shown positive effects in treating every single disease for which it has been studied.

Note: Many forms of curcumin are poorly absorbed. Look for a product that is confirmed bioavailable.

French Grape Seed Extract (*Vitis vinifera*): The oligomeric proanythocyanidins found in this botanical affect virtually every metabolic function in the human body.

Among its most researched anti-inflammatory and antioxidant properties are:

➢ Reverse cardiovascular disease, chemoprevention, anticancer and antimetastatic

➢ Improve glucose metabolism and reduce HbA1c

➢ Neuroprotective against beta amyloid plaque

➢ Speed wound healing

➢ Antibacterial against least 10 microorganisms, including MRSA

Andrographis (*Andrographis paniculata*): Little known outside of Asia, andrographis has been widely used in the Ayurvedic medical tradition, usage which has been validated by extensive Western research.

Andrographolides, the active ingredients, are a rare group of diterpenoid lactones, which have strong proven antimicrobial, anti-inflammatory and antioxidant effects. Andrographis is also a rich source of other nutrients, including well-researched antioxidant flavonoids and polyphenols.

Probably the most impressive overview of the pertinent research on andrographis and cancer comes from an international consortium of 19 scientists that confirmed andrographis' anticancer effects "on almost all types of cell lines" by:

➢ Neutralizing free radical damage and inflammation

➢ Stopping out-of-control cell lifespans

➢ Normalizing immune system response

➢ Stopping metastasis

➢ Promoting apoptosis

Its other most confirmed effects:

➢ Immunomodulation

➢ Antiviral, especially against several strains of influenza, including COVID-19 and HIV

➢ Antibacterial, including against *Staphylococcus aureus*

➢ Antitumor against a broad variety of cancers from at least five pathways

➢ Hepatoprotective

Berberine (*Berberis vulgaris*): I've conducted several studies on the alkaloid compound berberine, and I find that its ability to overcome chemoresistance is the most compelling. Specifically, it's effective in overcoming resistance to gemcitabine, not only in colorectal cancers, but also in pancreatic carcinomas.

Another impressive finding is that berberine helps lengthen telomeres, which has profound implications in promoting general longevity but specifically in treating and preventing all types of cancer.

Berberine has been proven effective in preventing metabolic syndrome, which is a cluster of disease factors including high blood pressure, elevated cholesterol, high triglycerides, high blood sugar and obesity that vastly increases the risk of diabetes and heart disease.

Berberine is also validated to:

➢ Promote weight loss

➢ Control blood sugars

➢ Enhance glucose regulation

➢ Activate AMPK

➢ Normalize lipids

➢ Reverse fatty liver disease

➢ Reverse congestive heart failure

Red Ginseng (*Panax ginseng*): This effective treatment for cancer, diabetes, erectile dysfunction and menopausal symptoms has been prized as an adaptogen in Traditional Chinese Medicine. Its active ginsenosides, also known as steroid-like saponins, are responsible for many of the herb's healing qualities. Some of the most important are Rb1 and Rb2 that fight inflammation, Rd and

Re that neutralize disease-causing free radicals and protect nerve cells, Rp1, Rg3 and Rh2 that attack cancer in a variety of ways and Rg1 that addresses the underlying causes of Alzheimer's disease and dozens more.

These major ginsenosides can be converted into rare ginsenosides by microorganisms in the digestive tract, making them far more potent healing agents.

Red ginseng's confirmed properties:

➢ Immune enhancement

➢ Anti-tumorigenic

➢ Relieves mental and physical fatigue (tonic and energizer)

➢ Treatment for Chronic Fatigue Syndrome and fibromyalgia

➢ Relieves chronic pain

➢ Calmative by reducing cortisol production

➢ Antidepressant

➢ Improve brain function, mental clarity and memory, decrease ARCD and cerebral ischemia

Greek Mountain Tea (*Sideritis scardica*): GMT's considerable healing properties are attributed to anti-inflammatory aromatic essential oils and antioxidant-rich polyphenols and flavonoids. These impressive anti-inflammatory compounds.

In today's science, Alzheimer's disease researchers are focusing research on GMT as a potential treatment and preventive for various forms of dementia.

Modern scientific research confirms GMT can:

➢ Combat Alzheimer's disease and cognitive decline

➢ Improve digestive health

➤ Lower blood pressure, reducing the risk of heart attacks and strokes

➤ Increase bone density

➤ Enhance immune function and prevent colds and flu

➤ Reduce anxiety and depression

➤ Reduce insulin resistance

➤ Promote weight loss

➤ Relieve joint pain

I prefer a product that combines Greek Mountain Tea with *Bacopa monnieri* for additional efficacy against emotional stress.

In my research, I have confirmed that some of these botanicals work synergistically.

Recommendations

➤ Curcumin with proven bioavailability with turmeric essential oil: 750 mg 2–3 softgel capsules daily for those who have been diagnosed with cancer

➤ Andrographis: 400 mg standardized at 20% yielding 80 mg of andrographolides, 400 mg 2–3 times daily

➤ French grape seed extract: tannin free, 400 mg soft-gel capsules, 2–3 daily

➤ Berberine with gamma-cyclodextrin: 250–500 mg

➤ Red ginseng with gamma cyclodextrin: 100 mg chewable tablet daily

➤ Greek Mountain Tea: capsule containing 450 mg daily, combined with 200 mg *Bacopa monnieri*

If you would like to investigate alternative medicine a bit more, and particularly the scientifically validated uses of these botanicals to treat a broad range of diseases, please feel free to contact my publisher (TTNPublishing.com)

We'll be happy to send you a free copy of the full book, *Alternative Medicine Works! Your Primer on Natural Medicine.*

References

For a deeper look at the science behind the supplements recommended in this book, please see:

Beat Cancer Naturally Now! The Five Most Powerful Natural Alternatives to Prevent and Treat Cancer. Ajay Goel, Ph.D., AGAF and Terry Lemerond. TTN Publishing, 2023.

Greek Mountain Tea: The Key to Mental Clarity and More. Terry Lemerond. TTN Publishing, 2023.

Discover Andrographis. Alex Panossian, Ph.D., Dr. Sci and Terry Lemerond, TTN Publishing 2023.

French Grape Seed Extract: Prevent and Reverse Cancer, Heart Disease, Diabetes, Alzheimer's and More. Ajay Goel, M.S., Ph.D and Terry Lemerond. TTN Publishing, 2023.

Red Ginseng: The Asian Heal All Herb. Jacob Teitelbaum. M.D. and Terry Lemerond. TTN Publishing. 2022.

Index

About the Authors

Dr. Ajay Goel

Ajay Goel, Ph.D., is Director of Epigenetics and Cancer Prevention at Baylor University Medical Center in Dallas, TX. He has spent 20 years researching cancer and has been the lead author or contributor to nearly 200 scientific articles published in peer-reviewed international journals and several book chapters. He is currently researching the prevention of gastrointestinal cancers using integrative and alternative approaches, including botanical products. Two of the primary botanicals he is investigating are curcumin (from turmeric) and boswellia.

Dr. Goel is a member of the American Association for Cancer Research and the American Gastroenterology Association and is on the international editorial boards of *World Journal of Gastroenterology* and *World Journal of Gastrointestinal Oncology*. He also performs peer-reviewing activities for almost 50 scientific journals, as well as serves on various grant-funding committees of the National Institutes of Health.

Terry Lemerond

Terry Lemerond is a natural health expert with over 55 years of experience. He has owned health food stores, founded dietary supplement companies, and formulated over 500 products to help people live healthier lives. A much sought-after speaker and accomplished author, Terry shares his wealth of experience and knowledge in health and nutrition through social media, newsletters, podcasts, webinars, and personal speaking engagements.

His books include *Seven Keys to Vibrant Health, Seven Keys to Unlimited Personal Achievement, 50+ Natural Health Secrets Proven to Change Your Life*, and his newest publication, *Discovering Your Best Health – How to Improve Your Health at Any Age.* Terry's weekly radio program, *Terry Talks Nutrition*, airs locally in Green Bay, Wisconsin Saturday and Sunday mornings at 8:00 a.m. CST, and is available online through his educational website at TerryTalksNutrition.com. His continual dedication, energy, and zeal are part of his ongoing mission—to improve the health of America.

KNOWLEDGE IS POWER,

ESPECIALLY FOR YOUR HEALTH!

Are you in search of a reliable, science-based resource for all your health and nutrition questions? Terry Talks Nutrition has you covered.

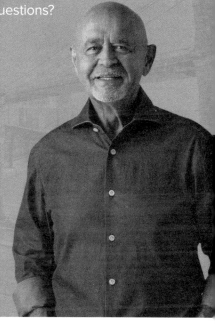

Connect with Terry to increase your knowledge on a wide variety of topics, including immunity, pain, curcumin and cancer, diabetes, and so much more!

READ

Visit TerryTalksNutrition.com today's latest and latest health and nutrition information.

LISTEN

Tune in on Sat. and Sun. 8-9 am (CST) at TerryTalksNutrition.com for a live internet radio show hosted by Terry! You can listen to past shows on the website or on your favorite podcast app.

ENGAGE

Connect with us on Facebook, where you can engage with other individuals seeking safe and effective ways to improve overall wellness.

WATCH

Check out our educational YouTube Channel to learn from the world's leading doctors and health experts.

Simply open your smartphone camera. Hold over desired code above for more information.

Get answers to all of your health questions at **TERRYTALKSNUTRITION.COM**

WELCOME TO

ttn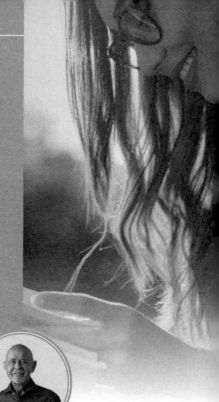
publishing

Are you ready to learn how anyone can use natural medicines, safely and effectively, to improve their health? You'll love TTN Publishing, my newest endeavor to bring you cutting edge research on powerful, health-supporting botanicals. I've coauthored numerous books with top alternative doctors from around the world to help you learn all you can about taking your health into your own hands. These educational books, supported by powerful scientific research, contain all the information you need to live a life of vibrant health.

In Good Health,
Terry Lemerond

ADDITIONAL BOOKS BY TTN PUBLISHING:

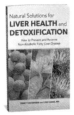 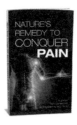 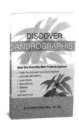 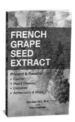 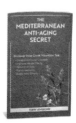 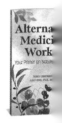

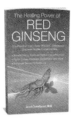 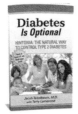 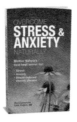 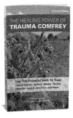 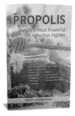 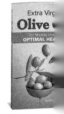

Get a copy for yourself and gift them to the people you care about!